I0481676

How To Be A Terrible Doctor

HOW TO BE A TERRIBLE DOCTOR

A 10 Step Manifesto of Commandments

Kolya K. Jaxson, MD

TITL Ventures

Copyright © 2018 Kolya K. Jaxson, MD
All rights reserved.

ISBN: 1983499862
ISBN 13: 9781983499869

TABLE OF CONTENTS

"Your appointment with life
is in the present moment.
The place of your appointment
is right here, in this very place."

Good evening. Or good morning. Or afternoon. Whenever it is you are reading this, your linear existence just improved exponentially. Why, you may ask?

Quite simply because, in your possession right here, right now, is a Holy Grail of sorts. A code crack, a life hack that strips away years or perhaps even decades of wasted time and effort in pursuit of perfection. You are reading the definitive guide for your quest to realize your ultimate potential. It is the blueprint, validated through art and science, the mystical and spiritual proofs of direct experience.

Befitting the sacred and solemn power of these truths, they are presented as a 10 Step Manifesto of Commandments. Like a vital organ, each step holds a unique character, a life force energy fueling its *raison d'etre*. But it is only in their synergistic integration that the parts beget the whole, and all possibilities yield to our preordained arrival and attainment of the coveted status: Terrible Doctor.

Let's begin our journey.

STEP #1: NEVER LISTEN
(TO OTHERS)

The true essence of perfection is unity. Completeness. An intact whole. Total tonal harmony. To this end, in order to attain your goal of becoming a Terrible Doctor, you must at all costs NEVER LISTEN. What does this mean?

Listening implies sharing, a fundamentally divisive endeavor. It is an affront to the fortress of your absolute certainty of all things. The physician alone, unique beyond compare, possesses the purest wisdom, nobility of intent, and functional expertise. Nothing within his personal or professional realm, or rather, any realm, exceeds his capable grasp.

Many factions will challenge you to hear their plaintive cries. Patients will offer their personal insights, as if your divine diagnostic powers were meant for input from the uncleansed masses. Pharmacists will plea to dilute the potency of your salves and elixirs, recipes beyond their mediocre intellects and indeed, supersed-ing the logic and limits of physiks and physiology.

Nurses, aye, they occupy a most special position in the hellish armada of striving tricksters and charlatans begging you to listen. For they serve as a sort of dual agent, pressing not only their own agendas but duly ad-vocating on behalf of their patients.

Why, the timid RN inquires, does the patient need IV fluids when, between vaping in the bathroom, they are consuming a 64-ounce energy drink from the local convenience store? When will you speak to the family member that has waited 4 hours for a word with you? Doctor, the patient has told me they wish to die. How can I possibly give chemotherapy?

The folly of these entreaties will be evident to the Terrible Doctor. You are being solicited. The first and foremost defense? NEVER LISTEN.

STEP #2: NEVER LISTEN (TO YOURSELF)

T he corollary or companion to our first Step may be, upon first glance, counterintuitive or seemingly irrational. Whereas NEVER LISTENING to others occupies the top position among the inviolable Steps and is patently obvious in its logic and intent, NEVER LISTENING to the self may require further explanation. Dear reader, allow me the privilege.

The arduous journey of becoming a Terrible Doctor is one of sacrifice, laser focus and near slavish dedication to an ideal. As illustrated in STEP #1, external forces of Evil will conspire against you. These visible villains are blatantly evident and typically easily identified so that appropriate counterforce measures may be deployed.

Into our awareness we must also bring a hidden foe: the self. With ninja like stealth this mute assassin will sabotage your quest with silent and deadly lethality, like neurotoxic gas poisoning your soul.

Don't let it. The *bourgeoisie* calls of hunger, thirst, fatigue, anxiety, fear, depression, instinct, compassion, and spirituality do not apply to you. As we must NEVER LISTEN to others, so too must we NEVER LISTEN to ourselves.

STEP #3: NEVER ENGAGE

To engage, what is this?

Engagement suggests an involvement, a participation in the affairs and psychic *milieu* of an alien other.

The path to this trap of entangled commitment may be sudden and complete or insidious and incremental. Guard against both.

As to the former, a typical trigger may be an event of great proportions, joyous or ruinous, unanticipated or predicted. Birth, death, cure, relapse and other momentous occasions are capable of flipping a switch and opening the floodgates of fellow feeling, bathing all parties in a common humanity previously unrecognized.

In contrast to this lightening bolt of change is the drip drip drip evolutionary erosion of water on stone, compounding over eons toward ever more entrenched bondage of souls.

Eye contact. A sympathetic smile or tear. A hug. Relaxed posture in a seated position. Seeking commonality of interests, goals and philosophies.

Like the proverbial tale of the camel's nose entering the desert tent, these small seemingly innocuous acts will open the door for larger clearly undesirable actions.

A general defense to either attack is the simple yet powerful maxim Lean Out.

The beautiful elegance of this approach is applicable to each individual domain bearing risk, and should be accordingly adapted.

In all matters, avoidance is best and most absolute. Absence will starve the seeds of engagement of the nutrients essential to growth. When physical presence can be averted, do so. Make a phone call if you must, or pass messages via third parties, ideally a lower level uninformed member of the care team, preferably non clinical.

When contact is unavoidable, hunker down. Imagine an impenetrable wall of protection shielding you from the seep of engagement into or out of your hallowed space. Stand. Look away. Maintain distance. Be parsimonious with time. Display no emotion. Limit questions and answers, and ignore when possible.

Stay the course.

STEP #4: SPEAK IN TONGUES

Befitting the exalted perch of the physician, there exists a *lingua par excellence* endemic to the tribe. Confounding in its intricacy, indecipherable to the commoner, the language of medicine remains largely inaccessible beyond its disciples, and perhaps a select few etymologists educated in the Greek-Latin canon.

Keep it so.

At every instance necessitating communication, be it verbal or written, use jargon. Doing so will serve several purposes, achieving many goals.

You will create confusion, uncertainty and embarrassment, allies that will serve as an emphatic parry to their advances.

You will at least maintain, and likely widen, psychic distance between yourself and the prospective interlocutor, dis-couraging their will to proceed.

You will delineate clearly and authoritatively superiority of cognition.

As perhaps the most essential fabric of culture, our language defines us, sculpting novel beauty and elegance from the crude stone of a shapeless mass. Each occasion involving choice of words affords the opportunity to throw into sharp relief your chiseled features and distinguish yourself, paying homage to ancestors past. Seize these moments. Embrace impenetrable complexity. Spread the WORD.

STEP #5: NEVER BE WRONG

Mistakes, flaws, errors, miscues, trip ups, oversights, flubs, bloopers, blots, blunders, bungles, weaknesses. What have these in common with ye?

Nothing.

As a purveyor and practitioner of medicine, anything less than The Utmost for Your Highest must be professionally inconceivable. In all aspects of your craft, material or ethereal, standards must never be compromised. Hence, *ergo reducio,* the taint of imperfection cannot be tolerated. Whether in word, deed, or other display, a vigilant defender will quash any notions of internal or external lack.

A singular driving repetitive monolog shall train the brain to program itself accurately, leading to proper thought, word and action. Like the mantras of Zen masters, a merciless mentality of "I AM ALWAYS

CORRECT" or some similar derivation will accomplish the deed.

Now then, is this to suggest that our lives will not be sullied by the presence of incompetence, neglect and indifference? Obviously, no. Indeed, the polluting smog of lesser creatures surrounds the rare air occupied by the physician. As such, inferior intellects and characters may divine their proximity as an association or attribution of weak to strong. You must vigorously correct these perceptions.

Whenever and wherever want, need or tragedy reside, blame others. Nurses. Patients. Phlebotomists. Speech therapists. Transport staff. Housekeeping. Radiology techs. Case managers. Insurance companies. Equipment. Weather.

These and an infinite number of additional contaminating particles must be deflected and will be, with forceful blame and focus on their inadequacies.

A most solemn final topic cannot be avoided. In your orbit you will comingle, often intimately, with members of the brotherhood, your medical colleagues. It is said that blood is thicker than water, and this much is true. Blood, the *anima vitae* that we all possess yet rarely can mix, demonstrates a crucial principle. Where compatibility exists, our common blood strengthens and invigorates, rejuvenates us. Otherwise, as is most typical, foreign blood diminishes and sickens us, and very well may be fatal.

Vet your "colleagues," assume malicious intent behind their actions, and when in doubt destroy them preemptively with blame as you would lesser opponents. THEY must be wrong, never you. Fratricide, while unpleasant, remains an indisputable necessity.

STEP #6: MORE IS BETTER

In the spirit of exceptionalism we heed the siren's call: See more. Do more. Be more. MORE more.

Like a perpetual motion apparatus set in play by a divine engineer, a culture of plentitude will often largely self sustain within proper circumstances. It is important to instill the principles and practices necessary to enable such conditions. I shall explain.

The common man will be shackled by concepts of prudence and restraint, notions anathema to our cause. So that one may tap into otherwise inaccessible dimensions, a sustained pistoling stream of golden resources at max flow is required to blast through the innumerable layers of resin shielding the nectar sweet manna we crave.

Why use one generic medication when three non-formulary will do? Why allow our sharp instruments to corrode with neglect at the behest of shameful DNR or palliative directives? Do we wish our streets to be teeming with the living dead, idle specialists yearning to line their pockets with the ill begotten fruits of bogus consults?

Nay.

Accept your mission with solemn intent and Choose Wisely, regularly and frequently. Do things for their own sake, and yours. Will to power, with disregard for calls of control or limits.

The forge of initial tracks may be taxing, as is the lot of the pioneer treading new terrain. With relentless obedience, the patterns will ingrain and begin to self regulate as agent, host and environment converge. Patients, after enough neglect, will stop calling offices and instead present directly to the Accident and Emergency Department. ED providers will forgo assessments, automatically launching a battery of tests and medications, limiting the possibility of diversion toward lower intensity services. Hospitalists will pull like a magnet those patients with a whiff of credible diagnosis into the labyrinthine muck of the hospital, and proceduralists of all cloths will penetrate the orifices of their subjects, preferably spanning over several days at a languid pace optimal for maximum self-satisfaction.

Be all you can be. Do all you can be. The choice is yours.

STEP #7: NEVER SHARE

This tenet has been alluded to in prior Steps, though only in an immature pupal stage of development. To birth its beautiful *imago* we must expound further.

Sharing {from the Olde English *scearu*--"division, part into which something may be divided,"} mocks our ideal of Totality. It diminishes and dilutes you and unjustly empowers the feeble minds, spirits and bodies of those desperate for vitality and wisdom.

Patients possessed by a ravaged psyche will seek to fill their empty tanks of resilience by attempting to pry from you aliquots of hope, empathy and personal anecdote.

Coding and documentation personnel will fruitlessly attempt to deduce an ICD-10 code from your terse illegible scribblings, where paper is present, or your cloned copy and paste electronic opus masterpieces. Encountering assured futility and frustration, they will issue Clinical Documentation Integrity Queries, as coercive and unjust an instrument as ever devised by the most oppressive and subjugating dictatorships, requesting, by various turns of the screw, "Clarification," "Specificity," and most odious of all, "Clinical Validity."

You will not relent. Furthermore, after a counterattack of disproportionate severity, your response will be most apt: ICD-10 code W51.XXXA: Accidental striking against or bumped into by another person, sequela.

A final example perhaps best illustrates the crucial concept of NEVER SHARING. Behold the travesty of Interdisciplinary Rounds (IDR.)

Ill conceived, a mutant bastard child of the most illegitimate origins, this rickety shack lays on a faulty foundation premised upon the maddening theory that fifteen disparate authors with incompatible languages shall, after thirty minutes in a poorly ventilated cramped room, compose Shakespeare. Malarkey!

A core practice underlying this fallacious theorem of course entails the sapping of physician time, energy and knowledge as he swims mightily to keep his head above the toxic humors conspiring to drown. The full frontal assault of IDR on physician dominion has become quite En Vogue.

Hold on. Don't let go. Let all parties know—You're never gonna get it (My Lovin'.)

STEP #8: BE ELUSIVE

A bsence makes the heart grow fonder. Your heart, of course, which is really the only one of significance and merit.

Exalted gurus reside solitary upon the highest mountaintops, their own self-sufficient masters of fate, privy alone to their wisdom and company, worthy heirs to the son of Judah, Onan.

It is not without effort that this Nirvana of solitude will be realized. Myriad obstacles and traps seek to enslave you into spheres of professional companionship. Of thus have we previously spoken, with Absolute Hell epitomized by the outrage that is Interdisciplinary Rounds, and its quest for concrete clinical intentions, dates of discharge and the like.

Make yourself scarce. At clinic, deploy barriers to ensnare the flaming arrows careening your way. Limit access to weekday only banker's hours, with lunchtime contact denied. Construct Byzantine policies for even the simplest tasks such as requesting appointments, re-filling medications, or obtaining test results. Perplexing telephone triage systems will often suffice.

At hospital, observe extremes of hour, making rounds long before dawn or long after dusk. Do not announce your arrival or departure, and most certainly do not communicate with anyone in your path. Blend in inconspicuously.

If paged, ignore. If persistently paged, also ignore. If relentlessly paged, respond with cheer, explaining that your pager battery died, your cell phone was out of range, or you were not told you were on call.

In charting, opacity rules the day. Leave no indications of a plan of care, lest attributable responsibility be assigned. Discard continuity, logic and clarity in communication. It will neutralize your scent and divert pursuant hounds off your trail.

Strive for truancy yet understand that visible invisibility, audible silence, and fluid evasiveness will achieve approximate equivalence.

STEP #9: INTERRUPT

The art of skillful interruption is crucial to your development as a Terrible Doctor, and serves as a force multiplier to the other Steps discussed thus far. It is also a watchman of sorts, which will judiciously guide you back to your True North when deviating off course. Should you be lulled, bullied or otherwise unwisely enticed to listen, engage, share or traverse other pitfalls, a sharp interruption will re-navigate.

Scientific studies show that physicians are generally able to listen to patient's stories for a median of 18 to 23 seconds before interrupting in some fashion. For the lackluster provider such a standard will suffice. The truly distinguished Terrible Doctor will far exceed in strength, rapidity and repetition any such plebian benchmarks.

Go on the offensive and strike with verbal pre-interruption, shutting down conversation before it starts and monologuing on whatever chosen topic suits your current fancy. Maintain a proper catalogue of ready to serve saws or gripes, ready to deploy at a moment's notice.

Interrupt physically, with body language and facial expressions that convey termination of signal from the transmitting other. As well, do not neglect to interrupt at length, drawing inspiration from political filibusters of lore. Your natural proclivities and training will determine your strengths as an interrupter of the sprinter, middle distance, or marathoner variety. Familiarize yourself with the techniques and advantages of each and strive for a well-rounded arsenal.

Certainly, do not limit this tool to patient subjects, though they be the primary recipients of your effort. Nurses will often require acute as well as chronic maintenance interruptive therapy. Prattling on about such trivialities as changes in status, abnormal vital signs, critical lab values, drug allergies and advance directives, you will need to co-opt them effectively.

You will.

STEP #10: AT ALL COSTS, DISREGARD COST

In healthcare there exists a troublesome banter perpetuated by frugal minded frumps of the dimmest order. This discourse, generally under the dubious suffocating blanket of "value," seeks to emasculate and impoverish proper pricing via a voodoo economic relationship between quality and cost.

It is a well-known truism since time immemorial that the price of a good or service is inextricably directly correlated to its worth. Free-range *chateaubriand* nourishes the elite for top Bitcoin, whilst the downtrodden ruminate on Grade D factory farmed chuck steak for rupees. So too must it be for healthcare expenditures.

Brand name pharmaceuticals and biologics should be prescribed under all circumstances in order to preserve the integrity of your reputation and the confidence of your patients. The rank stench of therapeutic substitutions, particularly with generics, must be subverted. DAW, commonly interpreted as "dispense as written," shall become known for its true message: "Do as per my will."

Medical imaging, with its piercing insights into the soul and anatomy of disease, is under continual assault by guidelines and prior authorizations. Whether for the healthy housewife with an obviously benign headache or the weekend warrior with a similarly trivial back strain, it is appalling to deny the reassurance implicit in an emergent cerebral or lumbar MRI scan.

For a mere few thousand dollars, pocket change for even the most penurious patient, you must insist that these tests be done. Warn all parties of the dire consequences of testing forgone, and document it. Freely employ Against Medical Advice verbiage as it relates to patients, and belittle and berate insurance company medical directors, cajoling them to come and assume care for YOUR patient.

When medical versus procedural interventions are argued as equivalent, endorse the latter. Spine surgery, knee arthroscopy, and cardiac catheterization well represent such choices. Fight the conservative cowards curtailing cost in the name of "evidence." Let the words of no less an icon than Theodore Roosevelt guide you:

"Get action; do things, be sane; don't fritter away your time; take a place wherever you are and be somebody; get action."

Get action. And always rack up a massive bill.

EPILOGUE

You have been given the Carpenter's tools to craft the masterworks that will distinguish your life as a Terrible Doctor. With confidence and determination, heed the words of Mark 16:15-16: "Go ye into all the world, and preach the gospel to every creature. He that believeth and is baptized shall be saved; but he that believeth not shall be damned."

Believeth.

Fin

ABOUT THE AUTHOR

Kolya K. Jaxson is a physician in New York. This is his first Manifesto.

ABOUT TITL VENTURES

TITL Ventures is a global lifestyle syndicate.

www.ingramcontent.com/pod-product-compliance
Lightning Source LLC
Chambersburg PA
CBHW071200220526
45468CB00003B/1094